AGING WITH GOOD HEALTH

A Simple and Complete Guide to Maintaining a Younger Body, a Sharp Mind, and a Fulfilled Spirit.

By

Ruben M. McDonald

AGING WITH GOOD HEALTH: A Simple and Complete Guide to Maintaining a Younger Body, a Sharp Mind, and a Fulfilled Spirit.

Copyright © by Ruben M. McDonald|2024. All rights reserved.

The publisher's content must be obtained prior to this material being copied or reproduced in any way. As a result, the information inside cannot be transferred, stored electronically, or preserved in a database.

No portion of the document may be reproduced, scanned, faxed, or stored without permission from the *publisher or author.*

AGING WITH GOOD HEALTH: A Simple and Complete Guide to Maintaining a Younger Body, a Sharp Mind, and a Fulfilled Spirit.

CONTENTS

- INTRODUCTION 5
  - Realizing How Important It Is to Age Healthily 6
  - Overview of The Guide...9
- PART 1: PERSONAL HEALTH 12
- CHAPTER 1 12
- DIET AND NUTRITION 12
  - The Role of Nutrition On Aging Well 24
  - Forming A Harmonious Diet Plan......................................32
  - Superfoods for Longevity 40
- CHAPTER 2 48
- FITNESS AND EXERCISE 48
  - Advantages of Frequent Exercise 49
  - Exercise Types for Various Age Groups...........................57
  - Creating A Fitness Program That Is Sustainable 67
- CHAPTER 3 77
- SLEEP AND REST...77
  - Importance of Quality Sleep 77
  - Suggestions to Improve Sleeping Habits..........................86
  - Techniques for Relaxation to Improve Rest 95
- PART II: MENTAL CAPABILITY..104
- CHAPTER 4 104
- INTELLIGENT HEALTH 104
  - An Understanding of Aging and Brain Health................104

    Activities and Exercises That Improve the Brain 118

    Methods to Improve Focus and Memory 127

CHAPTER 5 138

MENTAL HEALTH AND WELLNESS 138

    Resolving Anxiety and Stress 138

    Cultivating Positive Emotions 149

    The Value of Personal Links 160

PART III: SPIRITUAL FULFILLMENT 172

CHAPTER 6 172

MEANING AND PURPOSE 172

    Determining Meaning in Later Life 172

    Engaging in Meaningful Activities 182

    Inner Peace Through Spiritual Practices 191

CHAPTER 7 201

AWAKENING AND MEDITATING 201

    Merits of Conscience in Ageing 201

    Methods of Meditation for Quietness and Serenity 209

    Including Mindfulness in Day-To-Day Activities 218

CONCLUSION 227

RECAP OF KEY POINTS 227

ADDITIONAL ASSISTANCE 247

Books on Healthy Aging: 247

NOTES 248

INTRODUCTION

Aging is a common phenomenon that affects all facets of our life. Our bodies alter with age, our minds develop, and our life perspectives broaden. Even yet, there is some degree of control over how we age. We can approach aging with elegance, vigor, and fulfillment if we have the appropriate information, routines, and mindset.

This book, "Aging with Good Health: A Clear and Comprehensive Guide to Preserving a Younger Body, a Sharp Mind, and a Contented Spirit," is meant to be your travel companion.

Regardless of when you started considering your aging process or how far along you are in life, this guide is designed to give you useful tips, doable solutions, and motivational viewpoints to help you age effectively.

Realizing How Important It Is to Age Healthily

Why is it so important to concentrate on aging well? Our health and well-being have a tremendous impact on every part of our lives, so that is where the answer rests. We can live a more vibrant, contented, and meaningful life as we age if we put our physical, mental, and spiritual health first.

Physical Wellness: The cornerstone of a happy existence is a healthy physique. We may enhance our physical well-being and experience greater energy, mobility, and resilience by following a balanced diet, getting regular exercise, giving adequate sleep a high priority, and taking proactive care of any health issues.

Mental Agility: Throughout our lifetimes, our minds continue to grow and develop into immensely powerful tools. We can keep our minds active, creative, and emotionally healthy as we age by fostering cognitive health, practicing mindfulness, participating in brain-stimulating activities, and building emotional resilience.

Beyond the state of our bodies and minds, spiritual fulfillment gives our life meaning and depth. Developing our spiritual well-being enhances our inner world and promotes a sense of fulfillment and connection, whether via meaningful relationships, purpose-driven activities, spiritual practices, or deeds of compassion and gratitude.

Overview of The Guide

This handbook is organized into three primary sections, each of which addresses a vital component of aging healthily:

Physical Wellness: We explore fitness and exercise, nutrition and diet, and the value of rest and sleep in Part I. The foundation for a robust and resilient body as we age is laid by these essential physical health pillars.

Mental Agility: Part II examines methods for preserving mental acuity and emotional resilience as well as emotional and cognitive wellness. This area provides you with skills to maintain an active and healthy mind, ranging from stress-reduction strategies to brain-boosting exercises.

Reaching Spiritual Fullness: Ultimately, Part III explores embracing spiritual activities that uplift the spirit, developing mindfulness and meditation skills, and discovering meaning and purpose in life. For a comprehensive strategy to age gracefully and fulfilled, these facets of spiritual fulfillment are crucial.

You can apply the useful advice, fact-based analysis, anecdotes, and doable tactics included in each section to improve your everyday life. This guide has something to offer everyone who wants to age well, regardless of whether they want to start modestly with lifestyle modifications or proceed on a life-changing journey of self-discovery.

Within the next pages, we cordially urge you to investigate, acquire knowledge about, and welcome the opportunities that come with healthy aging. Let's travel together toward vitality, wisdom, and fulfillment—a trip that honors the richness of life at all ages.

PART 1: PERSONAL HEALTH

CHAPTER 1

DIET AND NUTRITION

Diet and nutrition are crucial to our general health and well-being, particularly as we get older. Our emotional fortitude, cognitive ability, and physical health are all directly impacted by the food we consume. We will dispel common misconceptions, examine the key elements of a balanced diet for aging individuals, and offer helpful advice for making wise food decisions that promote a full and active life in this in-depth investigation of nutrition and diet.

Recognizing Nutrition's Contribution to Aging

At any age, proper nutrition is the cornerstone of good health, but as we age, the significance of this aspect increases. Essential nutrients from a well-balanced diet maintain optimal body functions, extend life, and lower the risk of chronic diseases including diabetes, heart disease, and cognitive decline that are frequently linked to aging.

Crucial Elements for Optimal Aging:

Proteins: Essential for immune system support, tissue repair, and preservation of muscular mass. Lean meats, seafood, beans, nuts, and dairy products are examples of sources.

Good Fats: Omega-3 fatty acids, which are abundant in walnuts, flaxseeds, and seafood, are especially advantageous for lowering inflammation and promoting brain function.

Fiber: Helps maintain regular bowel motions, improves digestive health, and lowers the risk of heart disease. Legumes, fruits, vegetables, and whole grains are all great sources of dietary fiber.

Vitamins and Minerals: Sufficient consumption of vitamins (such as vitamin D and B vitamins) and minerals (including calcium, magnesium, and potassium) is necessary for immune system function, bone strength, and general health.

Drinking plenty of water

Although it is frequently disregarded, enough hydration is essential for preserving cellular function, promoting digestion, and controlling body temperature. Drink eight glasses of water or more each day, and make sure you eat meals high in water content, like fruits and vegetables.

Dispelling Myths Regarding Nutrition and Aging

There are a lot of false beliefs about aging and nutrition. Let's dispel a few widespread misconceptions and offer fact-based advice:

Myth: People over 65 require less protein.

Fact: Although the amount of protein required varies depending on factors such as muscle mass and activity level, older persons still need enough protein to maintain bone density, muscular mass, and general health. Eating meals high in lean proteins is good for you as you age.

Myth: Fats in general are unhealthy. True or false: Not all fats are made equally. Nuts, avocados, and olive oil are good sources of healthy fats that are necessary for hormone production, inflammation reduction, and brain function. A well-balanced diet ought to contain these.

Myth: Changing one's eating habits is too late.

Factual statement: It's never too late to start eating better. Making even little changes—like increasing the amount of fruits and vegetables or favoring whole grains over refined carbs—can have a big impact on one's health.

Useful Advice for Maintaining a Healthy Diet as You Age:

Emphasis on Whole Foods

Prioritize eating full, unprocessed meals including vegetables, fruits, whole grains, lean meats, and healthy fats. These nutrient-dense meals promote general health.

Consciously Consuming Food:

Eat carefully, take note of your body's signals of hunger and fullness, and enjoy every taste. Eating mindfully can reduce overindulgence and increase satisfaction from meals.

The balanced plate method

Try to arrange different food categories and colors on your plate. Every meal should include nutritious grains, colorful veggies, lean proteins, and a supply of healthy fats.

Maintain Hydration:

Water is your best beverage throughout the day. Alcohol and sugar-filled drinks should be avoided as they might cause dehydration and empty calorie intake.

Cut Back on Added Sugars and Processed Foods:

Reduce the amount of processed foods, sugary snacks, and beverages with added sugars that you consume. For sweetness, choose natural sweeteners like fruit or honey.

Make a Plan:

To make sure you have wholesome options available, plan and prepare your meals in advance. By doing this, you can lessen your reliance on potentially less nutrient-dense convenience foods.

Speak with a Certified Dietitian: See a qualified dietician if you have any special dietary questions or medical issues. They can offer tailored advice and suggestions depending on your particular requirements.

You may use nutrition to support healthy aging, preserve vitality, and improve your overall quality of life by adopting these ideas and practices into your daily life.

Actual Success Stories:

Maria's Road to Better Health: A Case Study

Maria, a 65-year-old retired woman, had low energy, weight gain, and joint problems. Maria noticed notable changes in her health after switching to a whole foods-based, balanced diet, frequent exercise, and enough water. She felt more alive and invigorated than ever after losing weight and building muscle. Maria's narrative effectively illustrates the profound influence that dietary and lifestyle modifications may have on aging.

Diet and nutrition are effective strategies for maintaining vitality, encouraging healthy aging, and improving general well-being. You may optimize your diet to support a vibrant and satisfying life at any age by learning about the importance of important nutrients, dispelling common misconceptions, and putting practical advice for healthy eating into practice. Keep in mind that you can significantly enhance your quality of life and health by making simple changes. Cheers to aging young at heart, taking care of your body and mind, and confidently and joyfully embarking on the journey of healthy aging.

The Role of Nutrition On Aging Well

Eating a healthy diet is essential to aging properly. Our bodies change as we age, and these changes may affect our metabolism, nutritional requirements, and general health. Making dietary decisions that promote longevity, resilience, and vigor requires an understanding of how nutrition affects aging.

Age-Related Nutritional Needs:

Calorie Requirements: As people age, their metabolism and activity levels may alter, resulting in a decrease in total calories needed, but the quality of those calories becomes more crucial. Make an effort to eat a diet rich in nutrients that offers necessary vitamins, minerals, and antioxidants.

Protein Intake: As we age, sustaining our immune systems, muscular mass, and strength depends on consuming enough protein. Make sure your meals contain lean protein sources including fish, chicken, lentils, and tofu.

Vitamins and Minerals: As we age, several vitamins and minerals become more important. Examples of these are calcium for strong bones, potassium for heart health, vitamin B12 for neurological function, and vitamin D for healthy bones. To satisfy these nutrient requirements, include a range of fruits, vegetables, whole grains, and dairy products.

Good Fats: Omega-3 fatty acids, which are present in walnuts, flaxseeds, and seafood, are good for the heart, brain, and inflammation. Incorporate sources of good fats into your diet while limiting trans and saturated fats.

Dietary Influence on Healthy Aging:

Sustaining Muscle Mass: Consuming foods high in protein and engaging in regular exercise help maintain muscle mass and strength, which lowers the risk of frailty and sarcopenia.

Bone Health: Consuming enough calcium and vitamin D maintains bone density and lowers the risk of fractures and osteoporosis.

Heart Health: Eating a diet high in fruits, vegetables, whole grains, and healthy fats can help lower blood pressure, improve cardiovascular health, and lower cholesterol.

Brain performance: Vitamins, antioxidants, and omega-3 fatty acids all contribute to the maintenance of mood stability, memory, and cognitive performance.

Immune System Support: The body's defenses against infections and illnesses are bolstered by a diet rich in vitamins and minerals and well-balanced.

Obstacles & Things to Think About:

Changes in Digestion: As people age, their appetite, digestion, and nutrient absorption may all change. Choose foods that are high in nutrients and simple to digest; if necessary, consider eating smaller, more frequent meals.

Hydration: Dehydration may be more common in older persons. Drink water to stay hydrated throughout the day, and eat meals high in water content, such as fruits and vegetables.

Drug Interactions: Certain drugs may interfere with the metabolism or absorption of nutrients. Seek advice from medical professionals or a certified nutritionist to minimize nutrient intake and handle any possible interactions.

Useful Advice on Nutrition for Healthy Aging:

Eat a Variety of Foods: Make sure your meals include entire grains, lean meats, healthy fats, and a rainbow of fruits and vegetables.

Portion Control: To prevent overindulging and preserve a healthy weight, pay attention to portion proportions.

Reduce Added Sugars and Sodium: Cut back on sweet desserts, snacks, and processed foods that are rich in sodium.

Cook at Home: To have more control over ingredients and cooking techniques, prepare meals at home with fresh ingredients.

Keep Up: Keep abreast of dietary standards and guidelines specifically for older persons, and modify your diet accordingly.

Because it promotes overall well-being, cognitive function, and physical health, nutrition is essential for aging well. You may improve your vitality, resilience, and quality of life as you age by being aware of your nutritional needs, choosing wisely, and developing healthy eating habits. Recall that proper diet, together with consistent exercise, enough sleep, and mental health, is a major component of healthy aging. Accept the ability of wholesome foods to uplift your body, mind, and soul, and relish growing older with vigor and meaning.

Forming A Harmonious Diet Plan
Maintaining optimum health, energy levels, and general well-being requires a balanced diet. You can feed your

body the vital vitamins, minerals, protein, carbs, and healthy fats it needs to perform at its peak by including a range of nutrient-rich foods in your meals. This guide will cover the essential elements of a well-balanced diet plan, offer helpful hints for organizing and preparing meals, and discuss techniques for introducing diversity and moderation into your eating routine.

Knowing the Macronutrients: Proteins: The building blocks of the body, proteins are necessary for immunological response, muscle repair, and hormone synthesis. Incorporate lean protein sources like fish, poultry, tofu, lentils, and nuts into your diet. Carbohydrates: Carbohydrates give the body and brain the energy they need to carry out daily tasks. Select complex carbs over processed carbohydrates and sweets, such as those found in whole grains, fruits, vegetables, and legumes. Fats: Heart health, cognitive function, and hormone balance all depend on healthy fats, which can be found in nuts, avocados, olive oil, avocados, and fatty seafood. Reduce your intake of processed and fried foods that contain saturated and trans fats.

Micronutrient Incorporation:

Vitamins: To make sure you're getting a range of vitamins, such as vitamin C, vitamin A, vitamin K, and B vitamins, include a variety of fruits and vegetables in your meals.

Minerals: Include foods high in calcium, magnesium, potassium, and iron, among other important minerals. These minerals can be found in dairy products, leafy greens, nuts, seeds, and lean meats.

Antioxidants: To shield cells from oxidative damage and promote general health, eat foods high in antioxidants, such as berries, dark leafy greens, nuts, and seeds.

Moderation and Portion Control: Balanced Meals: To ensure long-lasting energy and nutrition intake, try to incorporate a balance of healthy fats, proteins, and carbs in each meal.

Portion Sizes: To prevent overindulging, pay attention to portion sizes. Measure portions, use smaller plates, and be aware of your body's signals of fullness and hunger.

Eat a range of foods in moderation, including occasional indulgences or treats. To preserve the overall nutritional balance, balance indulgences with nutrient-dense meals.

Planning and Preparing Meals:

Plan Ahead: Give your weekly meal plans some thought, making sure to include a variety of foods and a balance of foods.

Grocery shopping: To make sure you have everything you need for wholesome meals, make a shopping list based on your meal plan.

Prepared Ingredients: To make meal preparation easier on hectic days, wash, cut, and portion ingredients ahead of time.

Cook at Home: To have more control over ingredients and cooking techniques, cook meals at home whenever feasible using fresh, complete items.

Drinking plenty of water

Water: Drink a lot of water throughout the day to stay hydrated. Restrict your intake of alcohol and sugary drinks as they can lead to overindulgence in calories and dehydration.

Looking for Expert Advice:

certified Dietitian: For individualized advice and suggestions based on your unique dietary needs, health objectives, and lifestyle, think about speaking with a certified dietitian.

The secret to promoting general health, energy levels, and well-being is developing a balanced nutrition plan. Your body can receive the vital nutrients it requires to survive if you prioritize eating meals high in nutrients, controlling portion sizes, exercising sensibly, and staying hydrated. You can create gratifying and long-lasting eating habits that promote a healthy lifestyle by organizing your meals, cooking them, and getting help from a professional when necessary. Accept the variety of meals that are available and relish the process of eating healthfully for maximum energy and well-being.

Superfoods for Longevity

Superfoods are foods high in nutrients, and full of antioxidants, vitamins, minerals, and other health-promoting substances. By including these foods in your diet, you can increase immunity, promote general health, and lengthen your life. In this article, we'll look at some of the best superfoods that are linked to longer lifespans and talk about how to include them in your diet to get the most health advantages.

Berries:

Blueberries: Packed with heart-healthy antioxidants called anthocyanin, blueberries also have anti-inflammatory qualities and are associated with better cognitive and cardiovascular performance.

Acai Berries: Rich in fiber and heart-healthy lipids, acai berries are a powerhouse of antioxidants that help lower oxidative stress and promote heart health.

Greens with leaves:

Kale: Rich in antioxidants, fiber, and vitamins A, C, and K, kale promotes immune system performance, bone health, and detoxification.

Iron, vitamin, and mineral-rich spinach support good blood circulation, mental clarity, and general energy.

Seeds and Nuts:

Walnuts: Packed with protein, antioxidants, and omega-3 fatty acids, walnuts promote heart and brain health as well as the reduction of inflammation.

Chia Seeds: Rich in antioxidants, omega-3 fatty acids, and fiber, chia seeds promote healthy digestion, stable blood sugar levels, and fullness.

Fish

Salmon: Rich in protein, vitamin D, and omega-3 fatty acids, salmon promotes heart, brain, and joint health.

Sardines: Rich in protein, calcium, and omega-3 fatty acids, sardines support cardiovascular health, bone health, and the decrease of inflammation.

Turmeric

The key ingredient in turmeric, curcumin, supports immunological, cognitive, and joint health with its strong anti-inflammatory and antioxidant qualities.

Legumes:

Lentils: Packed with protein, fiber, and folate, lentils help regulate blood sugar, the heart, and the digestive system.

Chickpeas: Rich in minerals, fiber, and plant-based protein, chickpeas aid with blood sugar regulation, digestion, and satiety.

Green Tea:

Green tea is high in catechins, which are antioxidants that help the immune system, metabolism, and heart health. It's also connected to longer life and better brain function.

Fruits:

Avocado: Rich in fiber, vitamins, minerals, and heart-healthy fats, avocados also promote satiety and skin health.

Pomegranate: Packed with vitamins and antioxidants, pomegranates support heart health, and brain function, and have anti-aging advantages.

How to Include Superfoods in Your Diet.

Smoothies: To make a nutrient-dense smoothie, blend berries, leafy greens, chia seeds, and a little green tea.

Salads: For a vibrant and wholesome lunch, top salads with avocado, kale, walnuts, and spinach.

Grain Bowls: For a well-balanced bowl, top whole grains with lentils, chickpeas, veggies seasoned with turmeric, and a sprinkling of almonds.

Fish Dishes: Try salmon or sardines seasoned with turmeric and served over quinoa or leafy greens.

Snacks: For a filling and healthful snack, try making your trail mix with dried berries or nuts and seeds. Superfoods are potent supplements to a balanced diet because they include a variety of nutrients that promote health, vigor, and longevity. You can provide your body with the vital nutrients it needs to flourish by including these nutrient-dense foods in your meals and snacks. Try out various superfoods, recipes, and meal combos to find scrumptious and nourishing ways to enhance your well-being and lengthen your life.

CHAPTER 2

FITNESS AND EXERCISE

Fitness and exercise are essential for preserving general health, vigor, and well-being. Frequent exercise not only keeps you physically fit but also improves your longevity, emotional stability, and cerebral clarity. This guide will cover the value of fitness and exercise, as well as numerous exercise options appropriate for different age groups and building blocks for a long-lasting fitness regimen that will benefit your health for the rest of your life.

Advantages of Frequent Exercise

Cardiovascular Health: Exercise lowers blood pressure, strengthens the heart, enhances circulation, and minimizes the risk of cardiovascular illnesses like heart attacks and strokes.

Strength Training and Flexibility Exercises: Strength training and flexibility exercises contribute to increased bone density, improved posture, improved mobility, and the development of muscle mass.

Weight management: A healthy body composition, weight loss, and weight maintenance are supported by regular exercise and a balanced diet.

Mental Health: Engaging in physical activity generates endorphins, which are happy-promoting neurotransmitters that also help lower stress, anxiety, and depressive symptoms.

Cognitive Function: Exercise lowers the risk of cognitive decline with age by improving cognitive function, memory retention, focus, and overall brain health.

Regular exercise can enhance the length, quality, and general patterns of sleep, which can lead to more restful and rejuvenating sleep.

Exercise Types for Various Age Groups:

Youngsters and Teenagers: Prioritize age-appropriate physical activities to enhance motor skills, coordination, and overall physical development, such as running, leaping, playing sports, and active play.

Adults: For general fitness and health maintenance, combine aerobic workouts (such as walking, running, and cycling), strength training (such as weightlifting, and resistance bands), and flexibility exercises (such as yoga, and stretching).

Seniors: Give special attention to exercises like tai chi, mild yoga, water aerobics, and low-impact strength training that enhance balance, coordination, and flexibility. Seek advice from medical professionals regarding tailored exercise regimens.

Creating a Long-Term Exercise Program:

Establish Achievable and Realistic Fitness Goals: Determine your present level of fitness, your interests, and your health.

Select Pleasure-Seeking Activities: Discovering hobbies and workouts you enjoy will help you stay motivated and faithful to your fitness regimen.

Take Your Time and Advance Gradually: To avoid injury and burnout, start with a tolerable intensity and length and gradually increase it as your fitness improves.

Adapt Your Exercises: To keep your workout interesting and push various muscle groups, mix up your program. Try out some new workout regimens, educational programs, or outdoor pursuits.

Plan Frequent Exercise Times: Make exercise a regular part of your weekly routine by blocking out particular hours for it. Strive to engage in a minimum of two strength training sessions per week, along with at least 150 minutes of aerobic activity at a moderate level.

Listen to Your Body: Pay attention to the cues that your body gives you, and modify your exercise regimen accordingly. Recovery and rest are crucial components of a well-rounded exercise regimen.

Drink lots of water before, during, and after exercise to stay hydrated and fuel your body. Consume a well-balanced meal that meets your energy requirements and offers the vital nutrients you need to heal and rebuild your muscles.

Including Exercise in Everyday Activities:

Driving Activatedly: For short trips, choose to walk, ride a bike, or take public transit rather than drive.

Take Breaks: If your profession or way of life is sedentary, take regular breaks to stand up, stretch, and move around.

Outdoor Activities: Take part in outdoor pursuits with your loved ones, like hiking, gardening, swimming, or sports.

Enroll in Clubs or Fitness Classes: To keep yourself motivated and meet new people while working out, take part in community events, sports leagues, or group fitness programs.

Fitness and exercise are essential elements of a healthy lifestyle that improve mental and physical health as well as general quality of life. You can experience a life full of vitality, strength, and resilience by adopting a regular physical activity schedule, selecting activities that are appropriate for your age and fitness level, creating a sustainable fitness program, and incorporating movement into everyday life. Exercise is a lifetime partner on your journey to well-being, so embrace the joy of movement and make it a part of every step, workout, and movement you take.

Exercise Types for Various Age Groups

For people of all ages, physical activity is essential because it promotes general health, fitness, and well-being. However, age, fitness level, and certain health issues can all influence the kinds of workouts that are appropriate and helpful. This guide will cover a variety of age-appropriate exercise options, from kids and teens to adults and seniors, emphasizing the value of age-appropriate physical activity for the best possible health results.

Youngsters and Teenagers (Ages 5–17):

Play and Active Recreation: Playing sports like soccer, basketball, and swimming, as well as recreational activities like running, leaping, and climbing, are beneficial for children.

These exercises enhance social connection, cardiovascular fitness, coordination, and motor skills. Structured Activities: To improve their strength, flexibility, agility, and teamwork, adolescents can take part in team sports, dancing classes, martial arts, gymnastics, or gymnastics. Strength Training: Supervised strength training with bodyweight exercises, resistance bands, or small weights can assist older adolescents (ages 14–17) grow their muscles, strengthen their bones, and support their general physical development.

Adults (Age 18–64): Aerobic Exercises: To increase cardiovascular fitness, endurance, and calorie expenditure, adults can participate in a range of aerobic exercises, including walking, running, cycling, swimming, dancing, or aerobics courses. Strength Training: Including strength training activities using resistance bands, machines, or free weights improves posture, increases metabolism, and lowers the incidence of sarcopenia, or age-related muscle loss.

Exercises for Flexibility and Balance: Including exercises for flexibility and balance, such as yoga, Pilates, tai chi, or stretching regimens, improves joint mobility and decreases the chance of falls and accidents. This is particularly significant as adults age.

High-Intensity Interval Training (HIIT): HIIT exercises are good for increasing metabolism, burning calories, and improving cardiovascular fitness because they alternate short rest intervals with high-intensity exercise bursts.

Seniors (65 and Over): Low-Impact Aerobics: To maintain cardiovascular health, joint mobility, and general fitness without putting undue strain on joints, seniors can participate in low-impact aerobic activities including walking, water aerobics, stationary cycling, or chair exercises.

Strength and Resistance Training: Maintaining muscle mass, enhancing bone density, and sustaining functional abilities for everyday living can all be achieved by incorporating mild strength and resistance training utilizing bodyweight exercises, resistance bands, or light weights.

Flexibility and Equilibrium: Balance-focused motions, yoga, and tai chi are examples of workouts that enhance stability, and coordination, and lower the risk of falls. Stretching regimens and other flexibility exercises help to preserve the joint range of motion and flexibility.

Functional Fitness: To preserve their independence and functional abilities, seniors might benefit from workouts that replicate everyday activities including walking, climbing stairs, lifting objects, and reaching high.

Prenatal Yoga and Pilates: These classes address the changing demands of the pregnant body, enhance flexibility, and encourage relaxation. They also emphasize gentle stretches, breathing exercises, and pelvic floor exercises.

Low-impact aerobics: Exercises that improve cardiovascular health without placing an undue strain on joints, such as walking, swimming, or stationary cycling, are appropriate for pregnant women of all trimesters.

Exercises for Strength and Stability: Exercises that target the pelvic floor, strengthen the core, and enhance posture can help reduce pregnancy-related discomfort and get the body ready for childbirth.

Exercises designed for particular age groups guarantee that people may get the most out of physical activity while lowering their chance of strain or injury. Strength training when necessary, organized play, and structured activities are beneficial for kids and teenagers. To maintain general fitness, adults can partake in a range of aerobic, strength-training, flexibility, and balance exercises. Low-impact aerobics, strength training, balancing exercises, and functional fitness are beneficial for seniors to maintain their independence and good aging. Exercises designed specifically for expectant mothers can help them stay healthy and support the physical changes that pregnancy brings about. Taking part in age-appropriate exercise encourages generations to commit to fitness and health for the rest of their lives.

Creating A Fitness Program That Is Sustainable

Establishing a sustainable fitness regimen is essential for long-term health, consistency, and enjoyment of exercise. In addition to assisting you in reaching your fitness objectives, a well-thought-out and balanced regimen improves your general health and quality of life. We will go over important ideas in this book to help you create a long-term, sustainable exercise regimen that will guarantee your success and well-being.

Establish Specific, Achievable Goals:

Establish Your Goals: Determine your fitness objectives, whether they are related to general health and wellness, muscle gain, increased endurance, or flexibility.

Be Measurable and Specific: Establish measurable, precise objectives for yourself, e.g., "I want to run a 5K in under 30 minutes" or "I aim to lose 10 pounds in three months."

Divide Objectives into Doable Steps: To keep track of progress and stay motivated, break down more ambitious goals into more manageable milestones.

Select Pleasure-Seeking Activities: Discover Your Interest: Choose workouts and pursuits that you look forward to and like, whether it's swimming, hiking, cycling, dancing, or group fitness courses.

Variety Is Essential: Mix up your regimen to keep things interesting and work for different muscle groups. Try novel exercises or vary your routines regularly.

Take Your Time and Advance Gradually:

Prevent Overtraining: In particular, if you're returning to exercise after a break or are new to it, start with a manageable time and intensity. As your fitness level rises, gradually increase the intensity, duration, and frequency. Pay Attention to Your Body: Observe your body's reaction to exercise and recovery. Between workouts, give yourself enough time to relax and recover to avoid weariness and reduce the chance of damage.

Combine flexibility, strength, and cardio Training: Cardiovascular Exercise: To strengthen your heart, burn calories, and increase your endurance, incorporate aerobic exercises like cycling, swimming, walking, running, or dancing.

Strength Training: To increase muscle strength, boost metabolism, and maintain bone density, use resistance training with weights, resistance bands, or bodyweight exercises.

Flexibility and Mobility: To improve flexibility, and joint range of motion, and lower the risk of injury, don't forget to incorporate mobility exercises, yoga, or stretching.

Plan Frequent Exercises:

The Secret Is Consistency: Make sure to prioritize and plan your workouts ahead of time, just like you would any other important appointment.

Allocate Time: Aim for two or more days of strength training that concentrate on your main muscle groups in addition to at least 150 minutes of moderate-intensity aerobic exercise each week.

Be Adaptable: Give yourself room in your calendar for unforeseen events or hectic days. Even shorter workouts or active pauses throughout the day can improve your general level of fitness.

Track Results and Make Adjustments as Required:

Monitor Your Development: To measure your progress, celebrate your accomplishments, and keep track of your activities, utilize activity trackers, fitness apps, or a workout journal.

Modifications and Challenges: To keep improving, periodically review your objectives, make modifications to your training regimen, and push yourself with heavier weights, more difficult workouts, or higher intensities.

Make rest and recovery a priority:

Rest Days: Give yourself time each week to enable your muscles to rest, recuperate, and heal. Active recuperation techniques like yoga, walking, and light stretching can help. Prioritize getting a good night's sleep to help with energy levels, muscle repair, and general well-being.

Nutrition and Hydration: Fuel Your Body: Keep a balanced diet that meets your energy demands and supports your fitness goals by including enough proteins, carbs, and healthy fats.

Hydration: To maximize performance, avoid dehydration, and promote recovery, drink plenty of water before, during, and after workouts.

The foundation of a lasting fitness program is balance, enjoyment, growth, and consistency. You can design a fitness regimen that fits your lifestyle and supports long-term health and well-being by setting clear goals, selecting activities you enjoy, starting slowly and building up to your desired level of fitness, combining cardio, strength, and flexibility training, planning regular workouts, tracking your progress, placing a high priority on rest and recovery, and providing your body with the right nutrition and hydration. Accept your fitness journey as a lifetime commitment to your well-being, vitality, and general standard of living.

CHAPTER 3

SLEEP AND REST

Importance of Quality Sleep

Good sleep affects our physical, mental, and emotional well-being and is essential for maintaining general health and well-being. Many people undervalue the relevance of consistently getting enough restorative sleep, even despite its importance. We'll examine the critical role that good sleep plays as well as the advantages it offers for optimum health and performance in this guide.

Physical Health Benefits: Regeneration and Healing: The body heals, regenerates, and repairs itself while you sleep. Good sleep promotes tissue healing, immune system performance, and general physical recuperation.

Heart Health: Sleep deprivation is associated with a decreased risk of stroke, hypertension, and heart disease. It supports cardiovascular health by assisting in the regulation of blood pressure, heart rate, and cholesterol levels.

Weight management: Sleep affects metabolism and the levels of the hunger hormones, leptin and ghrelin. Obesity, weight gain, and metabolic problems are linked to sleep disruptions.

Muscle Growth and Recovery: Getting enough sleep is crucial for the development and repair of muscles, especially following workouts or periods of intense physical activity. It supports the best possible sports performance and aids in muscular tissue restoration.

Hormonal Balance: Growth hormone, insulin, cortisol (stress hormone), and reproductive hormones are among the hormones whose production and control are impacted by sleep. Hormone balance is essential for general health and well-being.

Mental Health and Cognitive Function:

Brain Function: The ability to learn, solve problems, consolidate memories, and make decisions all depend on sleep. It improves brain clarity, focus, and cognitive function.

Emotional Regulation: Stable mood, stress reduction, and emotional resilience are all influenced by getting enough sleep. It lessens the likelihood of experiencing emotional problems, anger, depression, and anxiety.

Creativity and Productivity: Getting enough sleep promotes invention, creativity, and productivity. It improves one's capacity for mental creativity, problem-solving skills, and awake productivity.

Brain Health: Prolonged sleep deprivation is associated with a higher risk of neurodegenerative illnesses including Parkinson's and Alzheimer's. Restorative sleep lowers cognitive decline and promotes brain health.

Support for the Immune System: Immune System: A robust and healthy immune system depends on sleep. It strengthens the immune system, boosts immune cell production, and aids the body in fending against diseases and infections.

Inflammatory Response: Getting enough sleep lowers inflammation in the body, which is connected to several chronic illnesses including heart disease, diabetes, and autoimmune diseases.

Recovering from Illness: Getting enough sleep is essential for promoting the best possible healing, immune system performance, and general recovery during times of illness or injury recovery.

Ideas to Enhance the Quality of Your Sleep:

Create a Regular Sleep Schedule: Maintain a regular sleep and wake-up schedule every day, including on the weekends, to help your body's internal clock.

Establish a Calm Bedtime Routine: Read before bed, take a warm bath, practice relaxation techniques, listen to relaxing music, or do any combination of these things.

Optimize Your Sleep Environment: Make sure your bedroom is cozy and favorable to rest with a supportive mattress, cozy bedding, a pleasant temperature, and little light or noise.

Limit Screen Time: To avoid disrupting sleep, turn off electronics like computers, tablets, and smartphones at least an hour before bed. These gadgets generate blue light.

Mindful Eating and Drinking: Steer clear of large meals, coffee, and alcohol right before bed because these can throw off sleep cycles and reduce the quality of your sleep.

Frequent Exercise: Get moving regularly, but steer clear of strenuous exercise right before bed. Exercise helps to normalize sleep cycles and improves the quality of sleep.

Control Your Anxiety and Stress: Before going to bed, try some stress-reduction methods like yoga, deep breathing exercises, or mindfulness meditation to help you relax and quiet down.

A good night's sleep is crucial for general health, energy, and well-being. It is essential for immune system support, emotional control, cognitive function, physical health, and general life satisfaction. You may take advantage of the many advantages of getting enough sleep and improve your general quality of life by making healthy sleep habits a priority, setting up a peaceful sleeping environment, and implementing healthy sleep routines. Recall that getting enough good sleep is an essential requirement for living a long and healthy life, not an extravagance.

Suggestions to Improve Sleeping Habits

Although getting enough sleep is crucial for maintaining general health and well-being, many people have trouble falling asleep or have bad sleeping patterns. Creating a sleep-friendly atmosphere, sticking to a regular sleep schedule, and using relaxation techniques to encourage restorative sleep are all part of improving sleep patterns. We'll go through useful advice and techniques in this article to help you develop better sleeping habits and get a better night's sleep.

Create a Regular Sleep Schedule:

Establish Regular Bedtimes: Maintain a regular sleep and wake-up schedule, including on the weekends, to help your body's internal clock (circadian rhythm) work properly.

Steer clear of variations: Your body's natural sleep-wake cycle can be disturbed by irregular sleep habits, so try to avoid making big changes to your sleep routine.

Establish a Calm Bedtime Schedule: Relax Before Going to Bed: To tell your body it's time to go to sleep, take part in soothing activities. This can involve doing relaxation techniques, having a warm bath, reading a book, or listening to calming music.

Minimize Activities That Stimulate: Before going to bed, stay away from mentally taxing activities like strenuous exercise, using electronics, or watching TV because they can make it difficult for you to go to sleep.

Enhance Your Sleep Environment

Comfy Bedding: Invest in pillows and mattresses that will support your body and encourage sound sleep.

Room Conditions: To create the ideal sleeping environment, keep your bedroom dark, quiet, and cold. If needed, think about utilizing earplugs, blackout curtains, or a white noise generator.

Limit Screen Time: Because blue light from displays might interfere with your sleep-wake cycle, limit your time spent using screens (including TVs, laptops, tablets, and phones) at least an hour before bed.

Mindful Lighting: To tell your body when it's time to relax in the evening, use soft, dark lighting. Steer clear of intense brightness or bright overhead lights.

Maintain Good Sleep Practices:

Limit Alcohol and coffee: These substances might make it difficult for you to fall asleep and stay asleep, so avoid drinking coffee right before bed.

Avoid Large Meals: Large meals should be avoided right before bed because they can make you uncomfortable and interfere with your sleep.

Establish a Calm and Relaxing Ambience: Use aromatherapy, such as lavender essential oil, to establish a peaceful and comfortable environment in your bedroom.

Handle Stress and Anxiety: Before going to bed, try some stress-relieving methods to relax your body and mind. These include gradual muscle relaxation, deep breathing exercises, mindfulness, and meditation.

Create Healthful Sleeping Routines: Make Use of Your Bed to Sleep: Your bed should only be used for sleeping and private activities. To avoid associating your bed with awake, avoid using it for work, studying, or watching TV.

Keep Yourself Active: Throughout the day, take regular breaks from physical activity to improve the quality of your sleep and help you maintain a normal sleep-wake cycle.

Limit Naps: If you must take a nap during the day, do so for no more than 20 to 30 minutes, and try to avoid napping too soon before bed since this may disrupt your sleep at night.

Maintain a Sleep Journal: Keep a sleep journal to record your routines, sleep patterns, and any variables that might impact the quality of your sleep. This can be used to spot patterns and potential improvement areas.

If Needed, Seek Professional Assistance:

Speak with a Healthcare Professional: Even after forming healthy sleep habits, if you still have trouble falling asleep, see a doctor or sleep specialist for additional assessment and advice. Establishing positive sleep habits, practicing proper sleep hygiene, adjusting your sleeping environment, and developing a regular nighttime routine are all steps in the gradual process of improving your sleep patterns. You can improve the quality of your sleep, encourage peaceful and rejuvenating sleep, and take advantage of the many advantages of a good night's sleep for your general health and well-being by implementing these suggestions into your daily routine. Recall that getting enough good sleep is essential to leading a healthy lifestyle and that it should be given priority.

Techniques for Relaxation to Improve Rest

Effective strategies for encouraging greater sleep, lowering stress levels, and enhancing the general quality of sleep are relaxation techniques. You can tell your body and mind that it's time to relax by including relaxation techniques in your nightly routine. This will result in a more peaceful and revitalizing sleep experience. We'll look at a variety of relaxation methods in this tutorial to help you get better sleep and feel better overall.

Breathing Techniques:

Placing one hand on your abdomen while lying down comfortably is known as diaphragmatic breathing. Inhale deeply through your nostrils, allowing your abdomen to expand as air fills your lungs. As you slowly and fully exhale through your mouth, feel your belly drop. Repeat a few times, paying attention to the depth and pattern of your breaths.

4-7-8 Breathing exercises: Take a deep breath for four counts, hold it for seven counts, and then gently release it for eight counts. This breathing technique can help quiet a hyperactive mind and encourage relaxation.

PMR, or progressive muscle relaxation, is:

Stress and Relaxation: For a few seconds, tension the muscles in your toes, then release and fully relax them. Tension and release each muscle area as you move progressively up your body: your legs, abdomen, chest, arms, shoulders, neck, and face. As you let go of the tension in each muscle area, concentrate on the feeling of relaxation.

Meditation with mindfulness: Determine a comfortable sitting or laying position for focused attention. Shut your eyes and concentrate on your breathing or a single item, such as a flickering candle or a serene mental image. When your attention wanders, gently return it to your breath or the item, noticing any thoughts or sensations without passing judgment.

Body Scan Meditation: From your toes, slowly work your way up your body, focusing on any tense or uncomfortable spots. As you exhale, imagine these places becoming relaxed and releasing tension as you breathe into them.

Assisted Visualization:

Illustration: Imagine that you are in a calm and serene place, such as a mountain top, beach, or woodland. Visualize specifics such as the sights, sounds, scents, and feels of this peaceful area to stimulate your senses. Release any tension or concerns by allowing yourself to become fully submerged in this visual.

Positive Affirmations: Tell yourself things like "I am safe and at peace," "I am calm and relaxed," or "I release tension and embrace restful sleep."

Stretching and Yoga:

Easy Yoga Pose: Include easy yoga poses like Corpse Pose (Savasana), Child's Pose, Legs Up the Wall Pose, and Cat-Cow Stretch to help you decompress and release tension. Keep your breath deep and your actions deliberate.

Stretching Exercise: To increase flexibility and relieve tense muscles before bed, engage in a mild stretching practice. Stretching should be concentrated on the major muscular groups, such as the back, hips, legs, shoulders, and neck.

Aromatherapy:

Lavender Essential Oil: Put a few drops on your pillow or pulse points, or use it in a diffuser. The peaceful and relaxing qualities of lavender may help you sleep better.

Other Calming aromas: To create a relaxing environment that is favorable to rest, try other calming aromas like bergamot, cedar wood, or chamomile.

Including Relaxation Methods in Your Daily Routine:

Make regular use of one or more calming methods that you find calming as part of your nightly routine.

Dim the lights, turn down the volume, and remove any distractions to create a calm sleeping atmosphere.

Making relaxation techniques a habit will help you teach your body that it's time to wind down and get ready for sleep. Consistency is essential.

Relaxation methods are useful tools for lowering stress levels, encouraging deeper sleep, and enhancing the general quality of sleep. You can create a relaxing and sleep-promoting atmosphere by including deep breathing exercises, progressive muscle relaxation, guided imagery, mindfulness meditation, yoga, stretching, aromatherapy, or a mix of these techniques in your bedtime routine. Try out a variety of methods to see which one suits you the best, then reap the rewards of restorative sleep and improved relaxation.

PART II: MENTAL CAPABILITY

CHAPTER 4
INTELLIGENT HEALTH

An Understanding of Aging and Brain Health

It makes sense that as we become older, our interest in preserving ideal brain health will grow. The brain is a multifaceted organ that is essential to our overall well-being, emotions, and cognitive capacities. Maintaining mental acuity, memory, and quality of life requires an understanding of how aging affects the brain and what actions we may take to support brain health. The complexities of brain health and aging will be covered in detail in this guide, along with methods for maintaining a healthy brain as we age and variables affecting cognitive function.

The Changing and Difficulties of the Aging Brain

Neuroplasticity: The brain's extraordinary neuroplasticity allows it to evolve and adapt throughout life, in contrast to popular belief. But aging also brings with it certain adjustments and difficulties.

Structural Alterations: As we get older, our brains may become smaller and lose some of their neuronal connections, especially in regions that are involved in memory, processing speed, and executive function.

Changes in Cognitive Function: Aging can cause changes in cognitive function, including difficulties paying attention and multitasking, a loss of working memory capacity, and a slower rate of information processing.

Risk Factors: Genetics, lifestyle choices, health issues, and environmental factors are a few of the variables that may have an impact on age-related cognitive decline.

Enhancing Cognitive Function as We Age:

Healthy Lifestyle Decisions: Leading a healthy lifestyle has a major positive influence on brain function. This entails eating a well-balanced diet full of vitamins, omega-3 fatty acids, and antioxidants; avoiding bad habits like smoking and binge drinking; exercising frequently; effectively managing stress; and getting enough sleep.

Mental Stimulation: Keeping the mind busy and improving cognitive reserve can be achieved by partaking in mentally stimulating activities including reading, solving puzzles, picking up new skills, socializing, and taking up hobbies.

Exercise: Engaging in regular exercise enhances cardiovascular health and supports neurogenesis, or the creation of new brain cells, as well as brain function overall.

Brain-Healthy Diet: Eating a diet full of nutrients that strengthen the brain, like berries, nuts, seeds, leafy greens, fatty fish, and whole grains, can improve cognitive performance and stave off age-related cognitive decline.

Social Links: Retaining social ties and participating in activities with friends, family, and the community can stimulate the mind, offer emotional support, and create a feeling of community that is beneficial to brain health.

Cognitive training can assist in maintaining cognitive function and enhance cognitive resilience. These programs and brain exercises target memory, attention, and problem-solving abilities.

Stress management: Long-term stress can have detrimental effects on the health of the brain. Engaging in stress-reduction practices like tai chi, yoga, deep breathing exercises, or mindfulness meditation might boost brain resilience and lessen stress.

Routine Medical Exams: Conditions like depression, high blood pressure, diabetes, and high cholesterol that may affect brain health can be identified and treated with the aid of routine medical exams.

Enhancing the Brain with Nutrients and Supplements:

Omega-3 Fatty Acids: Flaxseeds, chia seeds, walnuts, salmon, mackerel, and other fatty fish are good sources of omega-3 fatty acids, which also lower inflammation, promote brain function, and guard against cognitive decline.

Antioxidants: Foods high in antioxidants, like dark chocolate, spinach, kale, berries (strawberries, blueberries), and kelp, can prevent oxidative stress and promote brain function.

Vitamin E: Rich in leafy greens, almonds, and seeds, vitamin E is an antioxidant that may help shield brain tissue from harm.

Vitamin B12: For optimal brain health and cognitive function, particularly in older persons, adequate quantities of vitamin B12, which can be found in animal products including meat, fish, eggs, and dairy, are essential.

Curcumin: A substance present in turmeric, curcumin possesses neuroprotective and anti-inflammatory qualities that may enhance brain function.

Supplements: Certain people may benefit from taking certain

supplements, such as omega-3 fish oil, vitamin B complex, vitamin D, or supplements that specifically improve cognitive function. Before beginning any new supplement regimen, it is crucial to speak with a healthcare provider.

Conditions and Difficulties Associated with the Aging Brain:

Alzheimer's disease, also known as dementia, is a common age-related neurodegenerative disorder marked by progressive cognitive decline, memory loss, and behavioral and functional abnormalities.

Mild Cognitive Impairment (MCI): This condition is characterized by observable cognitive changes that do not yet severely interfere with day-to-day functioning. In certain situations, it may be a sign of dementia.

Age-related vascular alterations can raise the risk of stroke and vascular dementia, as well as contribute to cognitive impairment. Examples of these changes include small vessel disease and decreased blood supply to the brain.

Additional Cognitive Obstacles: Deteriorations in attention, language, processing speed, and executive function are among the other cognitive obstacles that aging may bring.

Looking for Resources and Assistance:

Early Detection and Intervention: Improving results may come from early identification and treatment of cognitive abnormalities. Consult a healthcare provider for assessment and assistance if you or a loved one is experiencing notable cognitive changes or memory issues.

Supportive Services: For people with cognitive impairments and those who care for them, there are several supportive services and resources available. These include memory clinics, support groups, caregiver education courses, and local resources.

Legal and Financial Planning: It's critical for people with cognitive disabilities and their families to make plans, particularly those about legal and financial matters like estate planning, power of attorney, and advance directives.

Acknowledging the changes and difficulties that come with growing older, as well as putting measures into practice to support the best possible brain function and general well-being, are all part of understanding brain health and aging. A holistic strategy that incorporates brain-boosting nutrition, stress management, mental stimulation, social interaction, good lifestyle choices, and seeking help when necessary can help people maintain cognitive vigor and promote brain health as they age. A meaningful and vibrant life can be achieved throughout the aging process by adopting brain-healthy practices and remaining vigilant about brain health.

Activities and Exercises That Improve the Brain

Maintaining cognitive performance, encouraging neuroplasticity, and supporting general brain health all depend on engaging in brain-boosting activities and exercises. Engaging in these activities can activate various brain regions, improve neural connections, and support cognitive vigor and resilience. We'll look at many brain-boosting exercises and activities in this book that can help people of all ages become more intelligent, have better memories, and have higher cognitive abilities.

Brain Tears and Cognitive Difficulties: Brain teasers, Sudoku, logic puzzles, and crossword puzzles can test your memory, problem-solving abilities, and attention to detail.

Play card games like bridge or strategy-based board games like chess, Scrabble, or other games to improve your planning, strategy, and cognitive flexibility.

Acquire New Skills: To participate in lifelong learning, try studying a new language, painting, cooking, gardening, or playing an instrument. Acquiring new abilities fosters neuroplasticity and advances cognition.

Reading and Mental Imagery: Take up an interest in reading and use your imagination by reading novels, articles, or other literature. Imagination, creativity, and cognitive processing are all sparked by visualizing situations, people, and ideas.

Memory Exercises: Try improving your memory by memorizing passages of poetry or other texts, making lists, or playing memory games that test your recall skills.

Exercise and Mental Well-Being:

Regularly perform aerobic workouts including cycling, swimming, jogging, brisk walking, or dance. Aerobic exercise enhances brain blood flow, stimulates neurogenesis (the formation of new brain cells), and enhances cognitive performance.

Strength Training: Include activities that build muscle using body weight, resistance bands, or weights. Brain health and cognitive function are enhanced by strong muscles.

Exercises for Balance and Coordination: Activities that enhance proprioception, balance, and coordination—like yoga, tai chi, or dancing classes—benefit brain health by activating the parts of the brain responsible for motor control and coordination.

Meditation with mindfulness and relaxation:

Mindfulness Meditation: Engage in mindfulness meditation to develop present-moment awareness, lower stress levels, and enhance attention and concentration. Increased brain connectivity and emotional stability are two benefits of mindfulness.

Practice Deep Breathing: To help you relax, lower your anxiety level, and improve oxygen flow to your brain, practice deep breathing. Clear thinking and mental calmness are enhanced by deep breathing.

Progressive muscle relaxation, or PMR, is a technique that helps the body release tension and stress, which promotes mental clarity and relaxation.

Social Contact and Engagement: Socializing and Conversation: Take part in meaningful exchanges with friends, family, and neighbors through social activities and talks. Social interaction improves mental health, emotional stability, and cognitive performance.

Join Clubs or Groups: Get involved with clubs, associations, or organizations that are associated with your hobbies or interests. Engaging in group activities fosters cerebral stimulation, a sense of belonging, and social connections.

Volunteering: Take part in volunteer work or neighborhood service projects. Giving to worthy causes and serving others improves one's sense of purpose, well-being, and mental health.

Healthy Living Options:

Diet: Make sure you eat a healthy, well-balanced diet full of nutrients that are good for the brain, like antioxidants, vitamins, minerals, and omega-3 fatty acids. Healthy eating promotes cognitive vibrancy and brain function.

Enough Sleep: Set aside time for good sleep and create sound sleeping routines. Getting enough sleep is essential for brain health in general, memory consolidation, and cognitive function.

Stress management: Reduce chronic stress and promote brain resilience by putting stress-reduction strategies including mindfulness, relaxation techniques, physical activity, and time management into practice.

Promoting cognitive performance, maintaining brain health, and improving general well-being all depend on engaging in brain-boosting hobbies and workouts. You may enhance cognitive abilities, sharpen memory, preserve cognitive vigor across various stages of life, and optimize brain function by combining mental stimulation, physical activity, mindfulness practices, social engagement, and good lifestyle choices into your daily routine. Prioritize activities that stimulate and feed your mind for long-term cognitive well-being; adopt a holistic approach to brain health; and remain inquisitive and engaged.

Methods to Improve Focus and Memory

Crucial cognitive processes for day-to-day living, education, employment, and general well-being are memory and focus. Retention of information and focus can be impacted by a variety of factors, including lifestyle choices, mental exercise, and mindfulness techniques. We'll look at practical methods in this tutorial to help you focus better, remember things better, and use your cognitive abilities to their fullest.

Awareness and Mental Concentration: Practice mindfulness exercises to sharpen your attention and increase your sense of present-moment awareness. The mind can be trained to remain attentive and focused through deep breathing exercises, mindful eating, and mindfulness meditation.

Single-tasking: Prioritize one activity at a time as opposed to multitasking, which can decrease productivity and cause distractions. Set work priorities and give each task the time and attention it deserves.

Strategies for Retention and Mnemonics:

Visualization: Make better use of visual imagery to help you recall knowledge. Construct mental pictures or visual connections with the information you wish to retain.

To improve memory recall, associate new knowledge with ideas, pictures, or experiences that you already know. Establish significant linkages and correlations among concepts.

Chunking: Information should be divided into more manageable, smaller sections or divisions. To enhance memory recall, group similar items together.

Acrostics and acronyms: To help with memory recall, create phrases or sentences with the initial letter of each word corresponding to the information you wish to remember. These are known as acrostics or acronyms.

Use the loci approach, also known as memory palaces, to mentally picture a familiar place and link each location to a particular piece of knowledge. To memorize lists or sequences, this method works especially well.

Consistent Mental Excitation:

Play brain-twisting games and puzzles: Take part in puzzles, logic games, memory tests, Sudoku, crosswords, and brain-training applications. These exercises foster mental agility and test cognitive abilities.

Acquiring New Skills: To keep your mind sharp and involved, constantly acquire new abilities, hobbies, languages, or instruments. Acquiring knowledge increases neuroplasticity and improves cognitive abilities.

Optimal Lifestyle Practices:

Diet: Make sure you eat a healthy, well-balanced diet full of nutrients that are good for the brain, like antioxidants, vitamins, minerals, and omega-3 fatty acids. Nuts, seeds, leafy greens, berries, nuts, and fatty fish are foods that promote brain health.

Frequent Physical Activity: Physical activity helps the brain grow new brain cells, increase blood supply to it, and support cognitive performance. Exercises for strength, flexibility, and aerobic capacity should all be combined.

Enough Sleep: Set aside time for good sleep and create sound sleeping routines. Consolidation of memories, cognitive function, and general brain health all depend on sleep.

Stress management: Reduce stress by using time management, mindfulness exercises, physical activity, and relaxation techniques. Finding good coping mechanisms is crucial since long-term stress can impede concentration and memory.

Hydration: Make sure you stay hydrated by consuming enough water throughout the day. Concentration and cognitive function can be impacted by dehydration.

Arrangement and Time Management: Utilizing Planners and Calendars: Make use of planners, calendars, or digital apps to arrange assignments, appointments, due dates, and obligations. To efficiently manage your time, make notes and prioritize your responsibilities.

Task Breaking: To prevent feeling overwhelmed and to keep your attention on particular areas of the work, break up larger jobs into smaller, more manageable chunks.

Reduce the amount of distractions in your workstation or study location to create a distraction-free environment. Disable notifications, establish ground rules for disruptions and arrange your space so that it is calm and distraction-free so that you can focus.

Frequent Evaluation and Repetition:

Spaced Repetition: To review and reinforce material over time, use approaches using spaced repetition. Review sessions should be spaced out to improve long-term memory retention.

Active Recall: Put your newly acquired knowledge to the test by answering questions on it without consulting your notes or a textbook. This improves learning and helps with memory retrieval.

Organization, time management, mental stimulation, mindfulness exercises, memory techniques, and regular knowledge review are all important for improving memory and focus. You can maximize your cognitive function, enhance memory recall, increase focus, and succeed in many areas of your life by implementing these techniques into your everyday routine. To retain the best possible memory and focus throughout your life, keep in mind that consistency, practice, and a proactive approach to brain health are essential.

CHAPTER 5

MENTAL HEALTH AND WELLNESS

Resolving Anxiety and Stress

Common situations like stress and anxiety can have a big impact on one's physical, mental, and emotional health. Maintaining general health and quality of life requires knowing how to effectively manage and cope with stress and anxiety. We'll go over a variety of methods and strategies in this book to assist you in successfully managing stress and anxiety in day-to-day living.

Comprehending Anxiety and Stress:
Stress: Whether imagined or actual, stress is the body's reaction to perceived threats or problems. It sets off a chain reaction known as the "fight-or-flight" response, involving both physiological and psychological responses.

Anxiety: Anxiety is characterized by feelings of fear, trepidation, or worry over unknown or future occurrences. Physical signs including tense muscles, an accelerated heartbeat, and restlessness may appear.

Good Living Habits:

Frequent Physical Activity: To lower stress hormones like cortisol and encourage the release of endorphins, or feel-good chemicals, engage in regular exercise such as swimming, yoga, jogging, or walking.

Balanced Diet: Make sure your diet is healthy, full of whole grains, lean meats, fruits, veggies, and healthy fats. Steer clear of processed meals, sugar, and caffeine excess as these can make anxiety and tension worse.

Sufficient Sleep: Make sure you get enough good sleep by setting up a regular sleep pattern, a calming nighttime ritual, and a cozy sleeping space. Getting enough sleep is crucial for emotional health and stress reduction.

Mindful Eating: To practice mindful eating, observe your body's hunger signals, appreciate the flavors and textures of your meal, and abstain from emotional or stressful eating patterns.

Techniques for Stress Management:

Deep Breathing Exercises: To soothe the nervous system, lessen anxiety, and encourage relaxation, practice deep breathing exercises like diaphragmatic breathing or 4-7-8 breathing.

Progressive Muscle Relaxation (PMR): To relieve physical strain and encourage general relaxation, systematically tense and relax various muscle groups.

Mindfulness Meditation: Practice mindfulness meditation to develop emotional control, nonjudgmental acceptance, and present-moment awareness. Reactivity to stress is decreased and resilience is increased by mindfulness.

Yoga & Tai Chi: To relieve stress, increase flexibility, and encourage relaxation, take part in yoga or tai chi sessions. These forms of exercise integrate physical movement, breath awareness, and mindfulness practices.

Guided Imagery and Visualization: To lower anxiety and promote relaxation, use guided imagery or visualization techniques to conjure up images in your mind of serene, tranquil settings, like a beach or forest.

Cognitive-Behavioral Techniques: Cognitive restructuring involves questioning pessimistic cognitive patterns and substituting them with more pragmatic and optimistic ideas. Recognize and reframe cognitive distortions, such as black-and-white thinking and catastrophizing.

Problem-Solving Ability: To deal with pressures and obstacles in advance, and cultivate strong problem-solving abilities. Divide issues into doable steps, come up with possible fixes, and put plans of action into action.

Take part in Mindfulness-Based Stress Reduction (MBSR) seminars or workshops to learn how to combine mindfulness exercises with cognitive-behavioral strategies to lower stress, increase self-awareness, and strengthen coping mechanisms.

Social Links and Support:

Engage Others: Retain social ties with loved ones, friends, and those who can provide support. Seek emotional support, talk to someone about your feelings and concerns, and have meaningful interactions.

Join Support Groups: If you're interested in stress management, anxiety reduction, or mental health, think about attending support groups or counseling sessions. Make connections with people who have gone through comparable things to jointly discover coping mechanisms.

Healthy Boundaries: Establish limits in partnerships and obligations to control expectations, give self-care priority, and lessen stressors.

Organizing and Managing Time: Prioritize Tasks: To lessen overwhelm and efficiently manage workload, use time management strategies including prioritizing tasks, making to-do lists, and setting realistic goals.

Divide Larger jobs into Smaller phases: To reduce overwhelm and boost productivity, divide larger jobs into smaller, more manageable phases. Time for relaxing: Plan frequent pauses and leisure for hobbies, self-care, and relaxing. Strike a balance between times of relaxation renewal and productivity.

Looking for Expert Assistance: Therapy and Counseling: To investigate the root causes of stress and anxiety, acquire coping mechanisms, and obtain individualized support, think about seeking therapy or counseling from a mental health professional, such as a psychologist or counselor. Medication: In certain situations, using prescription drugs—such as antidepressants or anxiety medications—may help manage severe or ongoing anxiety symptoms. Seek advice from a medical expert regarding the best course of action for assessment and treatment.

A combination of cognitive-behavioral strategies, healthy living practices, stress management tactics, social support, time management, and, when necessary, professional assistance is required to effectively manage stress and anxiety. These techniques can help you manage stress better, develop coping mechanisms, strengthen emotional resilience, and generally improve your well-being daily. Recall that stress and anxiety management is a process that calls for perseverance, introspection, and a dedication to self-care.

Cultivating Positive Emotions

A satisfying life, mental toughness, and general well-being all depend on the cultivation of pleasant emotions. Good feelings promote mood and enjoyment, but they also strengthen relationships, improve physical health, and help people learn better coping mechanisms for difficult situations. We'll look at a variety of methods and techniques in this book to support you in developing and sustaining happy feelings in your day-to-day activities.

Recognizing Happy Feelings: Definition: Joy, thankfulness, love, contentment, amazement, inspiration, and optimism are examples of positive emotions. These feelings support a feeling of contentment, significance, and well-being in life.

Benefits: Developing happy emotions can help you feel less stressed, have a stronger immune system, be more resilient, have better mental health, be more creative, and have stronger social bonds.

Techniques for Fostering Happy Feelings:

Keeping a gratitude journal: Make a list of all the things you have every day to be thankful for, such as happy memories, deeds of kindness, or life's blessings. By concentrating on thankfulness, one can cultivate optimism and divert focus from negativity.

To develop present-moment awareness, acceptance, and nonjudgmental observation of thoughts and emotions, practice mindfulness meditation. Resilience and emotional control are improved by mindfulness.

Acts of Kindness: Show sympathy and kindness to other people. Feelings of happiness, empathy, and connection are increased when one helps others, volunteers, or engages in random acts of kindness.

Positive Affirmations: To combat negative self-talk and develop self-compassion, self-esteem, and a positive self-image, use positive affirmations, also known as self-affirmations.

Savoring Moments: Make a habit of savoring happy moments, beautiful moments, accomplishments, or little joys in life. Give your all to the present and recognize the good things that have happened to you.

Physical Activity: Exercise regularly to release endorphins, which are feel-good hormones that improve mood, reduce stress, and enhance general well-being.

Creative Expression: Investigate artistic, musical, literary, or crafty mediums. Self-expression, emotional release, and a sense of achievement are all facilitated by creative expression.

Positive Social Networks: Assemble a team of upbeat and encouraging individuals around you. Develop deep connections, spend time with those you love, and take part in enjoyable and uplifting social events.

Optimism & Positive Thinking: Instead of concentrating on issues or constraints, try to think positively and find solutions, chances, and possibilities. Having a growth mindset encourages resiliency and an optimistic view of life.

Laughter and comedy: Make time in your life to enjoy some comedy and laughter. Spend time with people who make you laugh, read hilarious novels or films, and discover the delight that comes from laughing's capacity to improve mood and lower stress levels. Conscious Emotion Management: Developing emotional awareness involves recognizing and accepting your emotions without passing judgment. Understand that all feelings—including negative ones—are a natural aspect of being human. Emotion Regulation Strategies: To effectively manage difficult emotions and foster emotional balance, practice emotion regulation strategies including progressive muscle relaxation, deep breathing, and cognitive reframing. Self-Compassion: Show yourself kindness and compassion, especially when things are tough or you're having setbacks. Engage in self-acceptance, self-compassion, and self-care to foster a supportive and encouraging internal conversation.

Good Living and Environment:

Healthy Lifestyle Decisions: To maintain a healthy lifestyle, give proper sleep, a balanced diet, frequent exercise, and stress reduction techniques top priority. A sound body nurtures a sound mind.

Declutter and Organize: Make your space clutter-free, orderly, and tidy to foster a feeling of peace, positivity, and order.

Reduce Adverse Influences: Reduce the amount of time you spend in unfavorable situations, poisonous relationships, or news sources that sap your vitality and exacerbate your bad feelings.

Introspective Techniques:

Everyday Reflection: Set aside time each day for mindfulness exercises or daily reflection, such as journaling, meditation, or silent introspection. Think back on the good times, things you've learned, and situations that have helped you grow.

Thankfulness Rituals: Make thankfulness a part of your everyday routine by sharing thanks with loved ones, reflecting on your gratitude before bed, or expressing gratitude before meals.

Developing good emotions is a life-changing process that includes deliberate activities, mental adjustments, and lifestyle decisions meant to promote happiness, thankfulness, forbearance, and overall well-being. You can develop a positive emotional state and reap the significant advantages of positivity on your mental, emotional, and physical health by integrating self-compassion, acts of kindness, mindfulness, gratitude, positive social relationships, and creative expression into your life. Accept optimism as your compass and treasure the times of happiness, progress, and connection that lead to a purposeful and happy life.

The Value of Personal Links

Human well-being is greatly impacted by social ties, which have an impact on everything from physical and mental health to emotional and mental well-being and general quality of life. Positive social connections that are formed and maintained can have a significant impact on our longevity, resilience, sense of belonging, and enjoyment. We'll look at the value of social bonds and their advantages for both people and communities in this tutorial.

Emotional Assistance and Welfare: Sense of Belonging: Social ties provide people with a feeling of inclusion and belonging, making them feel important, welcomed, and a part of a community. This feeling of community supports mental and emotional well-being. Emotional Support: During trying times, strong social networks can provide consolation, empathy, and understanding. Emotional resilience and coping mechanisms are enhanced when experiences, ideas, and feelings are shared with people you can trust. Cognitive Function and Mental Health: Decreased Risk of Anxiety and Depression: Healthy social connections and interactions lower the likelihood of anxiety, depression, and loneliness. A protective factor against mental health issues is social support.

Cognitive Stimulation: Social encounters, conversations, and activities improve mental acuity, memory, and mental dexterity. Participating in social activities enhances brain function and lowers the likelihood of cognitive aging. Advantages for Physical Health: Stress Reduction: Social interactions facilitate emotional expression, laughing, and relaxation, which in turn lowers stress levels. Supportive connections operate as a buffer between stress and the wellness of the body and mind.

Enhanced Immune Response: Stronger immune responses and higher general health outcomes are linked to positive social relationships. Immune response and disease resistance are improved by social support.

Longevity: Research continually demonstrates that those with strong social ties typically lead healthier, longer lives than people with fewer social supports. People who are socially connected have better health outcomes and reduced mortality rates across a range of age groups.

Improved Standard of Living:

Enhanced Happiness: Feelings of contentment, happiness, and life satisfaction are influenced by meaningful social interactions. Well-being is improved when experiences, joys, and achievements are shared with others.

Supporting Networks: Social ties give people access to resources, support systems, and chances for both career and personal development. Social capital and networking are essential for professional success, community involvement, and personal growth.

Good Social Influence: Exercise, a balanced diet, and self-care are examples of desirable behaviors that are encouraged by strong social interactions. Adopting healthy habits can be motivated, held accountable for, and encouraged by social ties.

Social Networks Throughout Life:

Childhood Development: Emotional growth, social skills, and self-esteem depend heavily on healthy social interactions and connections during childhood. Through their social interactions with peers and caregivers, children acquire the skills of empathy, communication, and dispute resolution.

Adolescent Support Systems: During times of identity discovery and transition, adolescents can benefit from the advice, validation, and peer acceptance that supportive social networks offer.

Relationships and Friendships for Adults: Adults flourish in social circles, romantic partnerships, and friendships that provide emotional support, intimacy, companionship, and common interests.

Socialization of the Elderly: Social ties are especially critical for older people because they support mental clarity, emotional stability, and a feeling of direction in life. In older populations, social involvement lowers feelings of loneliness and isolation.

Creating and Maintaining Social Networks:

Building meaningful connections and relationships requires the development of good communication skills, active listening, empathy, and emotional intelligence.

Social Activity Participation: Take part in clubs, hobbies, social activities, and community events that suit your values and interests. These environments offer chances to connect with people who share your interests.

Make the effort to connect with friends, family, neighbors, and coworkers by reaching out to them. Make the effort to keep in touch through frequent communication, plan social events, and preserve relationships.

Join Supportive Communities: Look for online forums, support groups, or communities that are relevant to your hobbies, objectives, or situation in life. These groups provide a feeling of understanding, community, and common experiences.

Give Back and Volunteer: Make a positive impact on your community by engaging in charitable work, deeds of kindness, or volunteer work. Contributing to the greater good cultivates altruism, social relationships, and a feeling of purpose.

Human well-being is largely dependent on social ties, which sustain mental, physical, emotional, and general quality of life. Positive social relationships need work, communication, empathy, and active involvement in communities and social activities. Building strong social ties throughout childhood, adolescence, adulthood, and beyond improves resilience, makes life more enjoyable, and makes society a better and healthier place overall. Accept the value of social interactions and give priority to establishing sustaining ties that promote both your well-being and the well-being of the people around you.

PART III: SPIRITUAL FULFILLMENT

CHAPTER 6

MEANING AND PURPOSE

Determining Meaning in Later Life

Later in life, there may be opportunities for introspection, personal development, and the pursuit of new goals and meanings. Transitions can happen to everyone; some people may retire or have an empty nest, while others might start new careers, follow interests, or make significant contributions to their communities.

This article will examine the significance of discovering a purpose in later life, methods for doing so, and the advantages it has for general contentment and well-being.

Identifying Your Later-Life Purpose: Definition of the Goal: A sense of direction, significance, and meaning in life is referred to as purpose. Finding the essential principles, objectives, interests, and contributions that provide purpose and fulfillment to life is part of it.

Significance in Later Years: Maintaining a sense of vitality, engagement, and fulfillment in older life depends on finding meaning. It gives one direction, a feeling of self, and inspiration for ongoing development and well-being.

Investigating Passions and Personal Values:

Spend some time reflecting on your values, convictions, areas of strength, and passions. Think about what pursuits, hobbies, or causes speak to you and make you feel fulfilled.

Life Review: Consider your prior encounters, successes, setbacks, and wisdom gained. Determine the important experiences, triumphs, and principles that have influenced your life's path.

Recognizing Contributions and Meaningful Activities:

Volunteering: Take part in volunteer activities that are consistent with your values and areas of interest. A sense of fulfillment and purpose can be obtained by making contributions to organizations or causes that are important to you.

Teaching and Mentoring: Whether through coaching, teaching, or mentoring, impart your knowledge, abilities, and experiences to others. It can be quite fulfilling to mentor younger generations or to give knowledge.

Creative Expression: Investigate artistic, literary, musical, or crafty mediums. Self-awareness, personal development, and a feeling of achievement are all facilitated by creative expression.

Participate in community-based clubs, events, or projects that support social justice, advocacy, or constructive change. It can be satisfying to be a part of a community and to change things.

Ongoing Education: Strive for both personal growth and lifetime learning. Enlarge your knowledge and skills by enrolling in classes, workshops, or seminars that pique your interest. Keeping Up Social Relationships: Maintaining social connections with friends, family, and peers is important. Support, company, and chances for development and connection are offered by meaningful social interactions and relationships. Joining Clubs and Groupings: Assemble social clubs, organizations, or groupings according to common interests or pastimes. Making friends with others who share your interests helps you feel like you belong and have a purpose.

Support Systems: Create strong systems of friends, mentors, and neighbors who will help and inspire you in your quest to discover your calling.

Accepting Change and Starting Over: The Opportunity of Retirement: Seize the chance to start over, explore, and follow passions you may have put on hold throughout your professional years after you retire.

Empty Nesting: Rekindle personal interests, pastimes, and fulfilling pursuits to welcome the empty nest stage of life.

Adapting to Change: Accept flexibility and change as a necessary component of life's journey. New experiences and interesting chances might arise from being adaptable and receptive to new encounters.

Finding a purpose later in life has advantages.

Greater Well-Being: Higher levels of happiness, contentment with life, and

pleasant emotions are linked to discovering a purpose in later life.
Sense of Fulfillment and Accomplishment: Encouraging meaningful activities and contributions makes one feel fulfilled and proud of their skills and achievements.
Better Mental Health: Having a purpose in life helps people feel more resilient mentally, less depressed, anxious, and lonely, and generally better mentally.
Physical Health Benefits: Research indicates that people who have a purpose in life typically live longer and

are more resilient to age-related obstacles.

Later-life purpose-finding is a transforming process involving meaningful interaction with life's possibilities, self-discovery, and exploration. People can find a purpose in life that enhances their quality of life and promotes overall fulfillment by thinking back on their values, passions, and contributions; doing meaningful activities; staying in touch with others; and welcoming changes with openness and optimism. Accept the chances for development, and relationships, and leave a lasting impression on both your own and other people's lives that later life brings.

Engaging in Meaningful Activities

For general well-being, fulfillment, and a sense of direction in life, meaningful activity participation is crucial. Engaging in activities that are in line with your beliefs, passions, and interests while also improving your mental, emotional, and physical well-being is considered meaningful. The significance of partaking in meaningful activities, methods for locating them, and the advantages they offer will all be covered in this guide.

Having an understanding of meaningful activities

Meaning: Engaging in meaningful activities is a great way to feel happy, fulfilled, and satisfied. Their alignment with your fundamental principles, convictions, and passions enhances your general welfare.

Categories of Purposeful Activities: A wide range of activities might be considered meaningful, such as creative endeavors, volunteering, social interactions, hobbies, educational opportunities, physical activities, and personal development activities.

How to Determine Your Passions and Values

Self-Evaluation: Identify your essential values, beliefs, strengths, and passions by spending some time introspecting about yourself. Think about the things that you enjoy doing that give you a sense of fulfillment and purpose. Establish your life's priorities, which may include things like spiritual fulfillment, personal development, relationships, health, and creativity.

Sync your actions with these top priorities.

Techniques for Taking Part in Important Activities:

After interests and hobbies: Whether it's painting, gardening, playing an instrument, cooking, or creating, set aside time for interests and hobbies that make you happy and fulfilled.

Volunteer and Give Back: Take part in community service or volunteer activity that is in line with your beliefs and causes that are important to you. Making a positive impact on other people's lives cultivates a sense of purpose and interpersonal relationships.

Investigate artistic mediums including writing, sketching, photography, dance, or music. Self-discovery, emotional release, and personal development are made possible through creative expression.

Engage in physical activities that you find enjoyable, such as yoga, hiking, dance, cycling, or team sports. Engaging in physical activity fosters a sense of success, well-being, and stress alleviation.

Learning Never Stops: Use online resources, workshops, seminars, and courses to continue learning throughout your life. Acquiring new abilities and knowledge promotes mental stimulation, self-actualization, and growth.

Social Engagement: By spending time with loved ones, joining organizations or groups, going to social gatherings, or taking part in group activities, you can cultivate meaningful relationships and social connections.

Setting Goals: Make significant plans for your development, your professional objectives, your physical and mental well-being, your artistic endeavors, or your social contributions. A purposeful goal-oriented approach gives drive and direction.

The advantages of participating in meaningful activities

Enhanced Well-Being: Happiness, contentment, and a sense of purpose in life are all influenced by meaningful activities. They give life fulfillment, direction, and significance.

Stress Reduction: Stress can be lowered and relaxation, emotional equilibrium, and resilience can be fostered by participating in activities you enjoy.

Better Mental Health: Engaging in meaningful activities increases one's sense of accomplishment, self-worth, and confidence, all of which contribute to better mental health. They also lessen loneliness, anxiety, and depressive symptoms.

Physical Health Benefits: Engaging in meaningful activities that promote physical activity, creativity, and social interaction can improve one's energy levels, longevity, and physical health.

Social engagement and connection with others are important aspects of meaningful activities that help build comradery, supportive connections, and a sense of belonging.

A great method to improve your well-being, sense of fulfillment, and quality of life is to get involved in meaningful activities. You can find happiness, meaning, and personal development by coordinating your actions with your beliefs, passions, interests, and priorities in life. Give priority to the things that make your life meaningful and fulfilling, whether they are volunteering, studying, producing, exercising, or interacting with people. Accept the path to a more fulfilling and fulfilling existence by embarking on a voyage of self-discovery and participating in worthwhile activities.

Inner Peace Through Spiritual Practices

It has long been understood that spiritual activities are effective means of fostering inner harmony, serenity, and a sense of oneness with something bigger than oneself. A vast array of customs, beliefs, and methods are included in these activities to foster the spiritual aspect of the human experience. In this book, we'll look at a variety of spiritual activities that might support you in discovering inner serenity, calmness, and a greater purpose in life.

Practice Mindfulness in Meditation: To develop present-moment awareness, deep relaxation, and nonjudgmental observation of thoughts and emotions, practice mindfulness meditation. Stress decrease, improved emotional control, and inner calm are all facilitated by mindfulness.

Breath Awareness: Pay attention to your breathing to help you center your focus in the here and now. Being aware of how you breathe helps you become more at ease and in control of your body.

Body Scan Meditation: Try body scan meditations to reduce stress, raise awareness of your body's various components, and encourage both mental and physical relaxation.

Together with breath awareness and attentive movement, practice yoga poses, or asanas, with tai chi. Yoga improves balance, flexibility, and inner serenity.

Tai Chi Movements: Practice Tai Chi, a gentle martial art that is well-known for fostering stress relief, relaxation, and the body's natural flow of energy, or Qi.

Prayer and Meditation: Praying aloud Pray to communicate with God, express your thanks, ask for wisdom, and develop a surrendered and connected sense of self.

Engage in contemplative practices by thinking back on spiritual lessons, holy writings, or philosophical issues that encourage introspection, awareness, and self-discovery.

Appreciation and Kindness:

Keeping a gratitude journal: To promote a happy outlook, an appreciation for life's benefits, and inner serenity, keep a gratitude diary in which you can record your blessings regularly.

Meditation on Loving-Kindness: Engage in mindfulness meditation (also known as Metta meditation) to develop compassion, empathy, and unwavering love for both yourself and other people.

Emotional health and inner tranquility are enhanced by this exercise.

Spend time outdoors by going on leisurely walks through parks, forests, or next to bodies of water. This is one way to connect with nature.

Experiencing nature firsthand fosters a sense of calm, wonder, and oneness with the natural world.

To strengthen your bond with the natural world and find moments of calm and tranquility, engage in the conscious study of its sights, sounds, and textures.

Stillness and Alone Time:

Silent Thought: Set aside time to engage in quiet introspection, contemplation, and reflection in a distraction-free, serene setting. You can connect to your inner wisdom and explore yourself in silence and solitude.

Digital detox: Make time for solitude, inner peace, and mindfulness by taking breaks from screens and gadgets.

Sacred Oaths and Traditions:

Creating Sacred Spaces: Set aside an area in your house or outside for spiritual activities, prayer, meditation, or introspection.

Ritual Practices: Take part in or design your rituals or ceremonies that pay tribute to your spiritual convictions, life changes, or goals.

Sangha and Community:

Spiritual Community: Join like-minded people in spiritual communities, associations, or events. A sense of community, belonging, and shared wisdom is fostered via sharing spiritual practices, insights, and experiences.

Participate in sangha activities: To strengthen your spiritual practice and relationships with others, take part in group meditation sessions, debates, or retreats. Sangha activities are gatherings of spiritual people. In-depth chances to develop inner harmony, serenity, and a stronger bond with the spiritual side of life are provided by spiritual practices. Adopting spiritual activities can nurture your soul, promote inner peace, and create a feeling of purpose and meaning. These practices can include mindfulness meditation, yoga, prayer, gratitude, connecting with nature, holy rituals, and community involvement.

Take a transforming journey towards inner peace and spiritual fulfillment by investigating and incorporating spiritual practices that align with your values, beliefs, and objectives.

CHAPTER 7

AWAKENING AND MEDITATING

Merits of Conscience in Ageing
Mindfulness is a modern practice with roots in ancient traditions such as Buddhism. It has gained popularity due to its deep benefits in enhancing mental clarity, emotional resilience, and well-being. With its many benefits that improve quality of life and promote healthy aging, mindfulness grows in importance as people get older. This tutorial will go over the particular advantages of mindfulness as we age

and how it enhances our general well-being.

Stress Reduction: Managing Transitions: Significant life transitions, like retirement, empty nesting, or health problems, are frequently associated with aging. People who practice mindfulness are better able to handle these changes with resilience, which lowers the tension and worry that comes with change.

Stress management: Deep breathing exercises and meditation are mindfulness techniques that help older persons manage stress more skillfully. These techniques also lower cortisol levels and foster a sense of inner peace and tranquility.

Enhanced Mental Health: Emotional Control: Mindfulness develops an understanding of feelings without passing judgment, which helps older people better control their emotions. This results in increased emotional balance and better mood stability.

Decreased Emotions of Loneliness: Mindfulness techniques promote inner awareness and connection to the present moment, which lessens emotions of loneliness and strengthens a person's sense of self and other connections.

Enhanced Cognitive Function: Brain Health: Research indicates that mindfulness may help older persons' cognitive abilities and mental health. Attention, memory, and executive function have all been linked to regular mindfulness meditation.

Prevention of Cognitive Decline: Studies have shown that mindfulness-based therapies can lower the incidence of age-related cognitive illnesses like dementia and Alzheimer's disease as well as assist prevent cognitive decline.

Benefits for Physical Health:

Pain management: By fostering calm and raising pain tolerance, mindfulness exercises like body scan meditation and mindful movement classes like yoga can assist senior citizens in managing chronic pain disorders.

Immune System Support: Research indicates that practicing mindfulness increases immunity, which improves general health and resilience to disease.

Enhanced Adaptability:

Adaptability: Being mindful helps one become more flexible and adaptive when handling life's obstacles. Those who practice mindfulness as an older adult are better able to deal with hardship, overcome failures, and keep a positive attitude.

Acceptance of Aging: Being mindful helps one develop self-compassion and a sympathetic attitude toward oneself, which in turn lessens self-criticism.

Improved Social Connections: Mindfulness practices cultivate empathy, attentive listening, and presence in interpersonal interactions, which lead to deeper, more meaningful connections with others. Relationships are enhanced and social ties are reinforced by this.

Community Engagement: Programs centered around mindfulness frequently include communities or group environments where senior citizens can interact, exchange stories, and encourage one another on their path toward mindfulness.

Higher Life Satisfaction: Mindfulness cultivates a sense of meaning, purpose, and satisfaction, which in turn raises one's overall quality of life. Seniors who engage in mindfulness practices express higher levels of well-being and life satisfaction.

Embracing the Present: Mindfulness enables people to live more satisfying lives by making the most of the present moment, appreciating events, and finding delight in routine tasks.

The mental, emotional, physical, and social facets of well-being are all positively impacted by mindfulness as people age. Older individuals can benefit from lower stress, better emotional and mental well-being, sharper cognitive performance, better physical health, greater resilience, stronger social ties, and an all-around superior quality of life by implementing mindfulness practices into their everyday lives. By practicing mindfulness, people can embrace life's changes, age gracefully, and develop a sense of contentment and serenity as they get older.

Methods of Meditation for Quietness and Serenity

For millennia, people have utilized the potent practice of meditation to develop inner calm, mental clarity, and a sense of tranquility. People can reap significant advantages for their mental, emotional, and spiritual health by practicing meditation. This tutorial will cover a variety of meditation practices that are intended to help people become more clear-headed and peaceful in their day-to-day lives.

Practice Mindfulness in Meditation: Keep Your Attention in the Here and Now: Focusing entirely on the here and now while avoiding passing judgment is the goal of mindfulness meditation. To practice mindfulness, pay attention to the sounds around you, your breath, or your physical sensations.

Mindfulness meditation is a useful tool for improving mental clarity, focus, and decision-making skills by calming the mind and reducing mental chatter.

Emotional Regulation: Mindfulness meditation enhances emotional balance by encouraging non-reactivity to thoughts and feelings, which lowers stress, anxiety, and overwhelm.

Breath Awareness Meditation: Deep Breathing: To soothe the nervous system and promote tranquility, engage in diaphragmatic breathing. Pay attention to how your body feels as air enters and exits it.

Breath awareness meditation facilitates the clearing of the mind by removing distracting thoughts, which leads to increased mental clarity, calmness, and relaxation.

Visualization Meditation: Guided Imagery: Picture quiet settings like a placid lake, woodland, or beach using guided visualization techniques. Feelings of calm and relaxation are improved by visualizing serene surroundings.

Clarity of Vision: Through mental blueprint-building and visualization of desired results, visualization meditation facilitates the clarification of objectives, desires, and intentions.

Relaxation Techniques: Body Scan Meditation: Progressive by methodically relaxing every body part, from head to toe, you can practice body scan meditation. With each breath, acknowledge any tension or discomfort and let it go.

Physical and Mental Clarity: By bringing awareness to physiological sensations, body scan meditation helps people relax physically, release tension from their muscles, and improve their mental clarity.

Practice Loving-Kindness Meditation to Develop Compassion: Sending positive thoughts, love, and compassion to oneself and other people is the practice of loving-kindness meditation. Recite affirmations like "May I be happy, may I be healthy, may I be peaceful" to develop compassion and calmness.

Emotional Clarity: A higher sense of inner harmony and tranquility is attained through loving-kindness

meditation, which promotes emotional clarity, empathy, and connection.
Reciting Sacred Words During Mantra Meditation When practicing meditation, pick a mantra or sacred word (such as "peace," "love," or "serenity") and repeat it aloud or silently. To relax and improve clarity, concentrate on the mantra's meaning and energy.

Spiritual Connection: The practice of mantra meditation fosters a calmer, more peaceful mind as well as a deeper spiritual connection.

Walking Meditation: Mindful Movement: When you walk, pay attention to every step you take, how it feels to move, and how you feel connected to the ground. Walk carefully and gently, focusing on your breathing and the environment around you.

Clarity in Motion: Walking meditation promotes mental clarity, stress reduction, and a sense of serenity through movement by fusing mindfulness with physical exercise.

Sitting in Silence for Silent Meditation: Focus on the here and now, as well as your body's and mind's experiences, while you sit quietly and away from outside distractions.

Profound Introspection and Inner Peace: As you connect with your true essence through silent meditation, you can experience heightened clarity and serenity as well as profound introspection and inner peace.

Powerful tools for promoting calmness and clarity in daily life are meditation techniques. People can reap significant advantages for their mental, emotional, and spiritual well-being by engaging in mindfulness, breath awareness, visualization, loving-kindness, mantra repetition, walking meditation, or silent contemplation. To improve mental clarity, foster inner calm, and develop a greater sense of serenity in all facets of life, incorporate these meditation practices into your daily practice.

Including Mindfulness in Day-To-Day Activities

Being present while paying attention to your thoughts, feelings, and environment without passing judgment is the practice of mindfulness, which has the power to transform. A higher sense of general contentment, lowered stress levels, enhanced focus, and enhanced well-being can result from incorporating mindfulness into daily life. This tutorial will look at doable strategies for incorporating mindfulness into several facets of your everyday life.

A Conscious Morning Routine

Be Aware When You Wake Up: Set an intention for mindfulness and take a few deep breaths to begin your day.

Mindful Hygiene Practices: Bring mindfulness to daily actions like brushing your teeth, taking a shower, or getting dressed. Refrain from grabbing electronics or indulging in distracting activities right away. Pay attention to the feelings, emotions, and tasks associated with each activity.

Eating without distractions: Engage in mindful eating by concentrating only on the act of eating away from devices such as TVs, phones, and computers. Take note of each bite's flavors, textures, and experiences.

Taste Every Bite: Eat more slowly, chew everything well, and enjoy the flavors of your food. Eating mindfully encourages better digestion, quantity management, and gratitude for filling meals.

Active Mindfully: Engage in Mindful Movement Whether you're dancing, walking, running, or doing yoga, move your body attentively. During an exercise, be aware of the emotions, feelings, and breath of your body. Stretching with awareness can help you relieve stress, increase your range of motion, and become more aware of your body's demands.

Techniques for Mindful Work: Single-tasking: As opposed to multitasking, concentrate on just one task at a time. Whether you're doing housework or work-related tasks, practice mindful single-tasking by devoting your whole focus to each activity.

In talks with coworkers, family, or friends, engage in mindful communication by speaking mindfully, listening intently, and giving your complete attention.

Take Mindful Breaks: Spread out your day's mindfulness activities into brief intervals. Stop, inhale deeply a few times, and focus your attention on your body, breath, and environment.

Take Mindful Walking Breaks: Whether at work or on the weekends, take mindful walks. Stroll at a leisurely pace, take in your surroundings, and concentrate on how each step feels.

Staying Aware During Daily Tasks: Cleaning with mindfulness is approaching home tasks with an awareness of every movement, feeling, and breath when organizing, cleaning, or tidying up.

By being present, paying attention to the traffic, and avoiding distractions like using a phone, drivers can cultivate mindfulness while behind the wheel.

Observe with Mindfulness During Your Evening Routine: Spend some time at night thinking back on your day. Without passing judgment, accept your feelings, experiences, and achievements.

Deep breathing, light stretching, or meditation are examples of mindful relaxation techniques that can help you unwind before bed to encourage sound sleep.

Resources & Apps for Mindfulness: Employ Apps for Mindfulness: Look into mindfulness applications that provide exercises, guided meditations, and daily reminders to practice mindfulness.

Study books about mindfulness: To improve your knowledge and everyday application of mindfulness, explore books and other resources on the subject.

It takes a journey of self-knowledge, alertness, and well-being to incorporate mindfulness into daily life. You can create a more thoughtful and satisfying existence by incorporating mindfulness into your daily duties, eating habits, exercise routine, morning routine, work tasks, breaks, and evening routine. You can also do this by using mindful apps and tools. Adopting mindfulness can improve your general quality of life and stress tolerance by helping you be more present, aware, and joyful in every moment.

CONCLUSION
RECAP OF KEY POINTS

We've looked at methods and techniques in this extensive guide to help people age gracefully and keep their health, intellect, and spirit intact. Let's review the main ideas discussed in this well-aging handbook.

Ernährung and Ernährung: Prioritize a diet that is well-balanced and full of whole grains, fruits, vegetables, lean meats, and healthy fats.

Drink plenty of water and cut back on processed meals, sugar, salt, and bad fats.

Prioritize obtaining nutrients from real meals and take supplements only if necessary.

Nutrition's Significance in Healthy Aging

As we age, optimal nutrition maintains the immune system, cognitive, and general health as well as energy levels. Prioritize consuming foods high in nutrients that offer vital vitamins, minerals, antioxidants, and phytonutrients.

Making a Diet Plan That Is Balanced: To guarantee a varied nutrient intake, plan meals with a range of food groups and colors.

Eat mindfully by observing your body's hunger signals, controlling your portion sizes, and eating slowly.

For individualized nutrition programs based on specific health concerns, seek professional advice.

Superfoods for Longevity: Because they are so good for you, include superfoods like berries, leafy greens, nuts, seeds, fatty fish, and legumes in your diet.

The antioxidants, fiber, omega-3 fatty acids, vitamins, and minerals included in these superfoods are crucial for healthy aging.

Workout and Health:

Take part in frequent physical activities such as aerobics, strength, flexibility, and balance exercises.

Together with muscle-strengthening exercises, try to get in at least 150 minutes of moderate-intensity activity per week.

Maintain an active lifestyle by minimizing sedentary behavior and introducing activity into everyday routines.

Regular Physical Activity's Advantages

Cardiovascular health, bone density, muscle strength, flexibility, and general physical function are all enhanced by regular exercise.

In addition, it helps with mood modulation, stress reduction, cognitive function, mental wellness, and sleep quality.

Different Exercise Types for Age Groups:

Individual needs and abilities should be taken into account while designing exercise regimens. This includes things like age, mobility, fitness level, and health issues.

Whether you want to walk, swim, practice yoga, dance, or strength train, pick pleasurable, sustainable, and safe activities.

Creating a Sustainable Exercise Program: Construct a well-rounded exercise program with elements for strength, flexibility, cardiovascular, and balance.

As you listen to your body and modify your workouts as necessary, progressively increase the intensity and duration of your sessions.

The significance of getting good sleep can be emphasized by making sure you follow a regular sleep schedule, setting up a calming bedtime ritual, and improving your sleeping environment. To enhance general well-being, happiness, cognitive performance, physical and mental health, and mood, aim for 7 to 9 hours of sleep each night.

Advice for Changing Your Sleeping Patterns:

Eliminate as much screen time and mentally taxing tasks as possible before bed.

Use calming methods to help you fall asleep, such as deep breathing, meditation, or light stretching.

Consult medical professionals about sleep issues or concerns for individualized treatment.

Methods of Relaxation to Promote Better Sleep:

To ease tension and anxiety and encourage relaxation, incorporate relaxation techniques into your everyday routine.

Methods like progressive muscle relaxation, guided imagery, deep breathing, and mindfulness meditation can improve the quality of your sleep.

Understanding Brain Health and Aging: Healthy lifestyle choices, lifelong learning, cognitive stimulation, and social interaction all contribute to maintaining brain health.

Preserve brain health by controlling long-term illnesses, cutting back on risk factors including smoking and binge drinking, and keeping a healthy weight.

Brain-Boosting Exercises and Activities:

To enhance mental agility and cognitive function, partake in brain-boosting activities including games, puzzles, reading, picking up new skills, and socializing.

Maintain mental stimulation and challenge to foster cognitive resilience and neuroplasticity.

Methods for Improving Concentration and Memory:

To improve memory and focus, use mnemonic devices, visualization exercises, repetition exercises, and organizational procedures.

To increase focus and attention span, keep your mind active, set priorities, reduce outside distractions, and engage in mindfulness exercises.

Handle stress and anxiety by using methods like progressive muscle relaxation, deep breathing, mindfulness meditation, and constructive coping mechanisms.

Effective stress management involves addressing underlying pressures, maintaining a healthy lifestyle, participating in enjoyable activities, and seeking out social support.

Developing Positive feelings: Through regular activities and mental adjustments, cultivate positive feelings like thankfulness, kindness, optimism, and resilience.

To improve general well-being and life satisfaction, emphasized relationships, growth, positive experiences, and self-care.

The value of meaningful relationships and social ties should be given top priority to promote mental health, lessen loneliness, and improve overall quality of life.

Keep up your social life, take part in neighborhood events, cultivate connections, and ask for help from loved ones when you need it.

Discovering a Higher Purpose in Later Life: Investigate your values, interests, and worthwhile pursuits that provide you with a sense of fulfillment, purpose, and contribution.

Motivation to Set Out on the Path to Healthy Aging

Choosing a good lifestyle, promoting holistic well-being, and developing a resilient and self-care mindset are all part of the transformational and powerful process of aging well. Aging brings with it special obstacles, but it also brings with it chances for wisdom, personal development, and a happy existence. Here are some words of inspiration and support to help you on your path to aging gracefully.

Accept Change as Growth: As we age, we naturally undergo events that mold our resilience, wisdom, and character.

Accept the age-related changes as chances for learning, development, and self-discovery.

Put Your Health First: Make healthy habits a priority for yourself by making nourishing food, consistent exercise, restful sleep, stress reduction, and preventive medical care a priority. Over time, small daily decisions can have a big impact on your well-being.

Maintain the well-being of your body, mind, and spirit:

Nurture your mind, body, and spirit as part of a holistic approach to well-being. Take part in pursuits that provide you with physical vigor, emotional equilibrium, cerebral clarity, and spiritual fulfillment.

Celebrate Your Journey: Recall and honor your accomplishments, significant anniversaries, and life lessons as you age. Every day is a chance to be grateful for what you have in life, to relish special times, and to consider your individual life story.

Continue to Learn and Remain Curious: Develop an inquiring mind and a hunger for information. To keep your mind active, read, take up new hobbies, acquire new skills, pursue creative endeavors, and look for intellectual stimulation.

Adopt Self-Care Practices: Give self-compassion and self-care top priority as they are vital to aging successfully. Develop healthy relationships with yourself and others by engaging in mindfulness, relaxation exercises, self-reflection, and gratitude.

Remain Physically Active and Interested: Continue to partake in things that make you happy, fulfilled, and socially connected. Engage in meaningful relationships with loved ones, volunteer work, hobbies, and community activities.

Develop Positivity and Resilience: Develop resilience by viewing setbacks as chances for improvement, adjusting to life's changes, and keeping a positive frame of mind. Remain grateful, keep your attention on what you can manage, and cultivate a resilient mindset.

Look for Assistance and Relationships: Create a solid network of family, friends, medical specialists, and local resources for support. Maintaining connections, getting help when you need it, and cultivating deep connections all enhance your well-being.

Accepting Age as a Blessing: View aging as a gift that offers wisdom, perspective, and a greater appreciation for life's richness by changing your viewpoint on it. Live with intention and purpose, embrace the present, and treasure your memories.

A personal and powerful decision, starting the journey to age well entails adopting healthy lifestyle practices, promoting resilience, developing holistic well-being, and discovering joy and fulfillment at every stage of life. Remember that every action you take to age gracefully is an investment in a lively, meaningful, and happy life. Stay positive and proactive. You can grow old with elegance and purpose since you are strong, wise, and capable.

ADDITIONAL ASSISTANCE

Books on Healthy Aging:

"Decoding Longevity: Investigating the Intersection of Science, Art and Culture in the pursuit of a longer life" written by Ruben M. McDonald.

"The Longevity Diet: Discover the New Science Behind Stem Cell Activation and Regeneration to Slow Aging, Fight Disease, and Optimize Weight" written by Valter Longo.

NOTES

AGING WITH GOOD HEALTH: A Simple and Complete Guide to Maintaining a Younger Body, a Sharp Mind, and a Fulfilled Spirit.

AGING WITH GOOD HEALTH: A Simple and Complete Guide to Maintaining a Younger Body, a Sharp Mind, and a Fulfilled Spirit.

www.ingramcontent.com/pod-product-compliance
Lightning Source LLC
Chambersburg PA
CBHW052145220526
45471CB00004B/1530